# Contents

# Prologue

Although there are various comprehensive books reinforcing the medical knowledge required to pass the MRCP written exams, there is surprisingly little information describing the overall strategy one should adopt.

A good analogy is that of a soldier: despite the fact he may win some battles by becoming a proficient fighter and user of weapons, he cannot realistically expect to continue doing so unless he familiarises himself with the surrounding terrain upon which the war is being fought. Likewise, to attain the MRCP diploma, you will be required to work hard on reinforcing the medical knowledge you accrued throughout medical school and clinical practice. In addition you must ensure that you familiarise yourself with the "terrain" of this exam.

The purpose of this guide is to act as that compass. It serves to take you through the terrain of the MRCP written exams where hopefully your hard work will shine through.

# What is MRCP?

MRCP stands for the Membership of the Royal College of Physicians. Once a candidate passes all three parts (parts I, II written and PACES) of their exam then they are elected to membership and awarded the MRCP diploma.

Part I consists of two 3-hour papers separated by a 1 hour break. Each paper comprises approximately 100 questions, totalling 200 questions in 6 hours. The question generally contains a stem which is then followed by five options, from which you have to pick the best one. Thus it is called best-of-five (BOF). A typical question example is as follows:

You are the cardiology CT1. An 82-year-old lady attends clinic with longstanding confirmed hypertension. Blood pressure today is 182/95. Her medication history includes amlodipine 10mg OD. Assuming she is fully compliant with her medication and this is a true reading what advice would you give her?

   A. Add doxazosin
   B. Add ramipril
   C. Ignore reading and reassure
   D. Add bendroflumethiazide
   E. Add bisoprolol

Each year MRCPUK dedicates a specific number of questions to each specialty to ensure coverage of all specialties. Recently this has been divided as follows:

| Specialty | Marks | Percentage of exam |
| --- | --- | --- |
| Cardiology | 15 | 7.5% |
| Clinical Haematology & Oncology | 15 | 7.5% |
| Clinical Pharmacology, Therapeutics & Toxicology | 16 | 8% |
| Clinical Sciences | 25 | 12.5% |
| Dermatology | 8 | 4% |
| Endocrinology | 15 | 7.5% |
| Geriatric Medicine | 4 | 2% |
| Gastroenterology | 15 | 7.5% |
| Infectious Diseases & GUM | 15 | 7.5% |
| Neurology | 15 | 7.5% |
| Nephrology | 15 | 7.5% |
| Ophthalmology | 4 | 2% |
| Psychiatry | 8 | 4% |
| Respiratory Medicine | 15 | 7.5% |
| Rheumatology | 15 | 7.5% |

The clinical sciences section is further subdivided as follows:

| | |
|---|---|
| Cell, Molecular & Membrane Biology | 2 |
| Clinical Anatomy | 3 |
| Clinical Biochemistry & Metabolism | 4 |
| Clinical Physiology | 4 |
| Genetics | 3 |
| Immunology | 4 |
| Statistics, Epidemiology & Evidence-based Medicine | 5 |

Part II written has a similar format but consists of three 3-hour papers. Papers 1 and 2 are held on day 1, separated by a 1-hour break. Paper 3 is held on day 2. Each paper comprises 90 questions, totalling 270 questions over 9 hours. Slightly more time is allowed for each question to accommodate for longer question stems. Part II continues the theme of focusing on the "major" medical specialties:

| Specialty | Marks | Percentage of exam |
|---|---|---|
| Cardiology | 25 | 9.3% |
| Dermatology | 13 | 4.8% |
| Endocrinology & Metabolic Medicine | 25 | 9.3% |
| Gastroenterology | 25 | 9.3% |
| Geriatric Medicine | 10 | 3.7% |
| Haematology | 13 | 4.8% |
| Infectious Diseases & GUM | 25 | 9.3% |
| Neurology | 25 | 9.3% |
| Nephrology | 25 | 9.3% |
| Oncology & Palliative Medicine | 13 | 4.8% |
| Ophthalmology | 4 | 1.5% |
| Psychiatry | 4 | 1.5% |
| Respiratory Medicine | 25 | 9.3% |
| Rheumatology | 13 | 4.8% |
| Therapeutics & Toxicology | 25 | 9.3% |

The specific breakdown of both exams is very important to our strategy and we will discuss this shortly.

## Who should sit MRCP?

Contrary to popular belief, candidates who attempt MRCP do not necessarily have to be aspiring physicians. In fact I have come across aspiring general practitioners; anaesthetists, radiologists and even a fully qualified pathologist who decided to retrain in general medicine!

However, the vast majority of candidates reading this guide will be aspiring physicians.

# When should I sit MRCP?

As soon as aspiring physicians overcome the hurdle of transitioning from medical student to real doctor, one of the first questions we ask ourselves is "When should I sit MRCP?".

Fortunately this difficult question has been made slightly easier by MRCPUK: "Part 1 is the entry-level examination accessible to doctors with a minimum of 12-months' postgraduate experience in medical employment."

This essentially means that the earliest you can attempt Part 1 is at the beginning (generally September) of foundation year 2 (FY2). Some deaneries and royal colleges go one step further and advise you to accrue more medical experience and wait until core medical training prior to attempting Part 1. This is evidenced at core medical training year 1 (CT1) applications where you'll find no additional shortlisting points awarded for an attempt or even a pass at the exam.

For me personally, the foundation years were the least demanding (hindsight is beautiful) in terms of workload and e-portfolio requirements so attempting in mid-FY2 isn't a bad idea at all. Be wary that if you attempt Part 1 in early FY2 you'll also be juggling CT1 applications. Multitasking never ends well for me...

A common concern with sitting Part 1 in FY2 is perceived lack of experience but personally, I never felt significant "shop floor time" was required for this initial hurdle. The exam can be considered as purely theoretical meaning a combination of familiarity with guidelines and repeating a relatively large number of practice questions should suffice.

If you're reading this having bested Part 1, take a breather and congratulate yourself first...but not too much. You're probably not going to like what follows.

# When should I sit MRCP Part 2?

One of the biggest regrets from Part 2 written candidates is taking a break after passing Part 1. Thus I'd recommend an attempt at Part 2 written immediately. I wouldn't worry about under-preparation because realise that the pass mark for Part 2 written is significantly lower than the previous exam and...you'll be fine.

All the work you did for Part 1 is half the battle trust me.

If you follow this guideline and work diligently then you may find yourself in the enviable position of having passed both written exams by the commencement of CT1.

However, if you're like me and wish someone gave you all this advice when you were a foundation trainee then do not despair. I passed all three MRCP exams within 10 months during CT1 so it's very achievable if you're willing to sacrifice some things.

## Where are the written exams held?

The UK exams are distributed country-wide and venues have included science
centres, churches, universities, hospitals and even rugby/football stadiums!

## How much do the exams cost?

Both UK exams cost £419 each. PACES costs £657.

# Why MRCP?

Good question. Why should I pay £1495 to sit these three exams? This figure does not include training websites, courses and resits!

For non-physicians, attempting MRCP part I demonstrates your holistic approach as a doctor. In particular, general practitioners may have had as little as 4 months of general medicine during FY1 followed by 6 months during GPVTS training before being expected to diagnose complex pathology on a daily basis. 10 months is not sufficient time to become adept at one medical specialty, let alone all of them!

For aspiring physicians, passing all three parts of MRCP is not an option. If you wish to progress to higher specialist training in any of the below 27 medical specialties then attaining the MRCP diploma is one of the requirements:

Acute Internal Medicine
Allergy
Audiovestibular Medicine
Cardiology
Clinical Genetics
Clinical Neurophysiology
Clinical Pharmacology & Therapeutics
Combined Infection Training
Dermatology
Endocrinology & Diabetes Mellitus
Gastroenterology

Genitourinary Medicine
Geriatric Medicine
Haematology
Immunology
Infectious Diseases & Tropical Medicine
Medical Microbiology
Medical Oncology
Medical Ophthalmology
Medical Virology
Neurology
Palliative Medicine
Rehabilitation Medicine
Renal Medicine
Respiratory Medicine
Rheumatology
Sport & Exercise Medicine

# How difficult is MRCP?

Just how difficult is MRCP? The answer to this question is dependent on who you ask!

In the old MRCP days of negative marking, when candidates answered a question incorrectly, they would've lost marks (as opposed to simply being awarded a zero nowadays).

Thankfully, negative marking no longer exists in MRCP but as you can see, pass rates for Part 1 and PACES remain low:

|  | UK Trainees | "Other" Trainees |
|---|---|---|
| MRCP Part 1, 2014 | 48.5% | 37.1% |
| MRCP Part 1, 2015 | 60.9% | 48.3% |
| MRCP Part 2, 2015 | 82.2% | 73% |
| MRCP PACES, 2015 | 61.6% | 36.4% |

Pass rates at first attempt, averaged over all three diets that year

MRCPUK state that candidates who did not declare their training details are reported as 'other trainees'. It's presumably fair to assume that this group largely consists of doctors who have either trained outside the UK, or are currently not within a formal training programme.

There are many reasons why 'other trainees' tend to perform less well than their UK counterparts.

Firstly, as this is a British exam, you would expect a larger emphasis on clinical conditions specific to UK clinical practice. This means alcoholic liver disease rather than malaria in the West of Scotland! Having said that, Part 1 still contains many 'weird and wonderful' conditions I've still not encountered in real life.

Another reason for the lower pass rate amongst 'other trainees' is that English may not be their native language. Certain words or phrases that UK graduates take for granted may not be so familiar for international graduates. After all, it makes sense that if you don't understand the question, you won't be able to answer it.

This language barrier becomes even more pronounced in the final clinical exam, PACES, where candidates are expected to take detailed clinical histories, explain investigations and results, break bad news, in addition to presenting entire cases to examiners under immense time pressure.

When referring to exams in general, scores can either be expressed as raw or scaled scores.

For example, a raw score of 70/100 can also be expressed as 70%. However if we want to compare the difficulty of this exam compared to its predecessor from last year then the raw score isn't very useful.

Let's imagine that we establish that compared to this year's exam, last year's was less challenging.

We introduce a scale from 0 to 300. If a mark of 72/100 last year is deemed equivalent to 70/100 this year by the experts then we assign the same scaled score (for example 220/300) to both marks. This is essentially what happens in the MRCP UK exams.

Instead of a percentage score, candidates are awarded an overall scaled score that ranges from 0 and 999. The current pass score for Part I is 528. The current pass score for Part 2 is 425.

Interestingly, Part 2 pass rates have been historically higher. This could be a result of the lower pass mark required but could also reflect survivorship bias – only candidates who have passed Part 1 are eligible to attempt Part 2 written.

Instead of becoming discouraged from attempting MRCP, I hope you'll use all this data to your advantage. One thing's for sure – MRCP isn't easy!

In conclusion, hopefully I've answered how difficult is MRCP? And remember that no matter how impressive they may be, all the registrars and consultants you work with were in your shoes at some point during their careers.
We were also apprehensive, and uncertainty followed us constantly like a dark cloud above our heads. Numerous consultants told me that failing multiple times prior to

success wasn't all that unusual and it certainly isn't a reliable indicator of clinical ability.

Part of the battle is having confidence in your own abilities and not comparing yourself to other people. Impostor syndrome is very common amongst medics and I'm quite sure all doctors experience this at some point in their lives.

After all, you've all passed medical school, which is a great achievement in itself.

# The difference between attempting and passing

Whilst revising for Part I, I consulted various registrars and consultants hoping for pieces of wisdom but I was frequently disappointed. Some were only concerned with finishing the ward round. Others chuckled about the number of times they had to re-sit the exam, which did not help my nerves at the time! A few just dismissed the exam as easy - in hindsight they were right but I'm looking at the exam from a completely different angle today.

I was adamant on finding a solution as I think most candidates enter the exam without a plan.

One of the most useful conversations I had was with my educational supervisor at the very beginning of CT1. He advised: "You must think about MRCP when you eat, sleep and work. Failing is not an option and you shouldn't 'attempt' an exam. You should aim to pass because if you don't, you set yourself back 3 – 4 months." He continued: "You end up losing confidence, dignity and you end up lining the pockets of those who charge extortionate exam fees."

The exam fees alone were a deterrent from failing.

My educational supervisor was right and based on his advice I went on to achieve the MRCP diploma in 10 months.

The sooner you attain Part I, the quicker you can attempt Part II written. This will enable you plenty of time to prepare for PACES. If you attain the MRCP diploma early, you can then concentrate on strengthening your applications for ST3 with additional publications, presentations, teaching and quality improvement projects. Moreover you may wish to use your time effectively by acting up as a medical registrar during CT2.

# Resources: practice makes perfect

By surviving medical school you have already proven your ability to memorise vast amounts of information. This automatically qualifies you as capable of passing Parts I & II written!

Every student has a slightly different study technique and this can range from rote learning to memory palaces to mind maps. However MRCP is an unusual exam in the sense that if you asked ten doctors for advice regarding resources for Part I, almost all of them will point you in the direction of practice questions.

Reading long guidelines can only take you so far and can become terribly dry. If you prefer textbooks then I would recommend *Essential Revision Notes for MRCP by Dr Philip Kalra* and the *Oxford Handbook of Clinical Medicine*.

If you study like your humble author then I recommend several question banks.

Question banks mentally place you in the clinical situation and can be very useful in the exam and also in clinical practice. It is more realistic than reading from a textbook and simulates the exam format well. Attempting the question stem followed by a 5-minute light reading session on the answer or the relevant guideline consolidates the information in your mind.

The question bank I recommend above the others is *Passmedicine* because it's relatively inexpensive and still boasts over 2,300 questions which I wasn't able to exhaust. The questions were high quality but I found them not to mimic the exam's format as closely as the others. However the explanations were excellent and followed guidelines to the letter which can be useful for the exam.

For Part I, I would also recommend *Onexamination*. There are rumours that 5% of the actual exam is based on questions in this bank! Personally I felt the questions were much more similar to the exam than *Passmedicine*. However the explanations were slightly short at times and I found myself having to drudge through NICE guidelines frequently.

The third popular question bank amongst my peers was *Pastest*. Personally I would not recommend them based on their questions bank. However, I would recommend them for their less well-known video and slide-show lectures.

They contain numerous video or slideshow lectures (by senior registrars and consultants in their fields) on each specialty taking you through their thought processes when tackling various questions. This is a very useful resource to maintain your sanity after doing a few hundred questions...

For Part 2 written I would recommend one book: *Rapid Review of Clinical Medicine for MRCP Part 2 by Dr Sanjay Sharma*. In my opinion, this book is very readable and Dr

Sharma takes you through every case as if you were on his consultant ward round. Although the format is not always BOF like in the exam, you should be familiar with the format by now! In this book, hundreds of patient cases are discussed, followed by investigation results and then thought provoking questions.

This mimics the Part 2 Written exam very well and you should familiarise yourself with common investigations including CXR, ECG, and interpretation of a wide collection of blood tests. If you have time to understand rarer investigations such as myocardial perfusion scans or PET scans then I'm impressed! However your return on investment is likely to be very low and chances are you won't use your new found knowledge in clinical practice unless you become a cardiologist or respiratory physician!

The following are the same question banks you may wish to use for Part II:

| Resource | Cost | Number of questions | Best for: |
|---|---|---|---|
| Passmedicine | £30 for 4 months or £40 for 6 months | 2,300 | Good explanations and direction to guidelines |
| Onexamination | Ranges from £82 for 2 months to £133 for 7 months | 3,300 | Similar format to exam style |
| Pastest | £99 until upcoming diet or £165 until the diet after | 5,000 | Excellent video and slideshow lectures |

## The main difference between Part I & Part II written

Although Parts I & II written have a similar format in the sense both exams are
BOF, there are some major differences.

If you have prepared adequately you will complete Part I with time to spare. You may even have time to go through every single question again in both papers if you have the stamina.

However in Part II written, even if you have prepared well, finishing on time is an achievement! The question stems are generally twice to three times as long as their counterparts from Part I. There are also numerous investigation results to analyse, all taking up previous minutes.

As a result, I would suggest setting yourself a time limit when tackling questions, as your Part II exam approaches.

# Thought process

When doing practice questions, memorising the answers to specific questions is never going to be enough. Firstly, although the MRCP written exams consist of 200 or 270 questions apiece, the question bank from which they are taken from are in excess of 30,000 questions. The chances of success using memorisation alone are very slim.

A better option is to attempt the full practice question, whilst imagining that you are in the clinical scenario. Attempt the question to the best of your ability and then check your attempt against the best answer. Regardless of whether you answered correctly or not, you should still read the explanations to ensure that your thought process is correct.

If I guessed every question blind-folded I would still expect to get 20% of the marks!

# Mixed Category Revision

Another important concept to consider is mixed category revision. Although there is nothing fundamentally wrong with setting up your revision by specialty when you are doing background reading, it is best to answer practice questions from an unknown category. Let me explain.

If the question stem consists of a patient who presents with breathlessness then this could relate to a cardiovascular, haematological or respiratory condition. In the case that you know it is a cardiovascular condition, you will have an unfair advantage during practice. This will then place you at a disadvantage in the actual exam.

# Time allocation

One of the main reasons why candidates fail is because they fail to allocate their time effectively. If you recall the number of marks each specialty is allocated you will understand that not all specialties are equal. In Part I, clinical sciences is worth 25 marks whilst only 4 marks are allocated to geriatric medicine. This is of utmost importance when deciding how much time you are planning to allocate to each specialty.

To work out how much time you have for each specialty you need to know how many hours you have left to study. Knowing you have 50 days until the exam is not that useful if you are holding a busy MAU job with 2 upcoming sets of nights and weekends.

Therefore to get a better idea you need to know how many hours you have.

If you have 50 days before the next diet and you are planning to revise for an average of 2 hours per day then you should divide the total number of marks in the exam by the total number of hours you have. If you were studying for Part I in this example then 100 hours divided by 200 marks means you can afford to spend 0.5 hours per mark of the exam. This means you can afford to allocate 7.5 hours of revision time to cardiology, 4 hours to psychiatry etc.

With this example, this means that even if you wish to become a gastroenterologist you should spend no longer than 7.5 hours of revision on this specialty.

That doesn't sound like a lot of time but you must be disciplined. Otherwise you may find at the very end of your revision that you have left haematology completely uncovered! Of course this is only rough guidance and you may wish to increase or decrease your allocation to each of your areas depending on your strengths and weaknesses.

It is important to reiterate that 50 days may sound like a long time for a multiple choice exam. However even in a 1 in 7 rota you only have 6 free weekends! To put that into perspective, your maximum study time is only a few hours after work and those 12 weekend days. If you factor in long days and night shifts then your time is even less. Do not forget to factor in rest time too and look after yourself.

If you are approaching the exam date with very little time then I recommend spending your time on the specialty that offers most points first. For example if you have clinical sciences and psychiatry uncovered but you only have 2 days left, I would recommend spending all your time on the former. The probability of you encountering questions on clinical science is statistically much higher.

# High yield facts & pattern recognition

With stocks and shares a high yield alone does not necessarily qualify the holding as a winner. You may have to consider why the stock or share is yielding such a high dividend - perhaps the business is sinking and is desperate for investors? We also need to consider other aspects such as dividend cover etc.

Thankfully exams are much simpler!

Memorising so-called high yield facts will definitely increase your return on investment. Taking cardiology as an example: a common scenario in the exam is that of the prolonged QTc interval on the ECG. If you spend 30 minutes memorising the main causes such as low electrolytes, various fancy drugs and the genetic conditions your ROI is likely to be very good. Contrast that with attempting to memorise all the different hepatitis C genotypes and we know how inefficient the latter approach is.

It is well known that cramming and superficial learning in this way is not useful in the long term but you will be surprised how much more clinical knowledge you have gained and retained by revising this way.

*Passmedicine* has a good application called the *Knowledge Tutor* which fires a quick series of short high yield questions at you. You can easily answer 100 of them in less than an hour if you don't read the explanations - this is assuming you are looking to quickly test your knowledge as you are approaching the end of your studying.

Another interesting aspect of the exam is pattern recognition. Just as you develop a more "natural" ability to read ECGs the more experience you have the same applies for this exam.

For example in the case of neurology, if the question consists of an overweight female patient who has come to your clinic with a headache then one of your top differentials should automatically be benign intracranial hypertension. If the question supplies extra clues such as papilloedema then you can be even more confident.

One word of warning though - you should still strongly consider the possibility of other diagnoses such as venous sinus thrombosis or intracerebral haemorrhage.

A good general rule to remember is that in Parts I & II, every piece of information is there for a reason. So if the same lady came to A&E following a head injury then it is probably not BIH!

# Variety

Candidates often underestimate the number of hours they need to study to pass Parts I & II. This is probably the second most common reason for failing after poor time allocation.

Although everyone's threshold for concentration varies it is safe to assume that you will need a break eventually. Some people will need more breaks than you and others will need fewer.

Part I is especially challenging for doctors on busy rotas (which is essentially every medical trainee). During this journey you should never be too hard on yourself or feel alone – understand that nobody wishes to study after a hospital shift regardless of how keen or motivated they are. Not to mention that leaving the ward on time is the exception rather than the rule. Then you have the weekends, long shifts and nights on a busy rota.

So it is fair to say that one of the attributes of the successful MRCP candidate is grit and determination! Embrace the difficulty of studying for postgraduate exams whilst holding a demanding job and remember that anything worth having never comes easy.

This is where I feel the importance of variety becomes paramount in the face of all these obstacles. When motivation is lowest at 7pm on Tuesday night and you find yourself trying to get through 50 practice questions and their dry explanations. Instead, here is what I suggest.

If you can afford it I would recommend signing up to all three practice question sites. Say you decide to allocate 2 hours of study time every night after a typical 9am - 5pm shift. Split this into 3 separate blocks of 40 minutes each. For the first block (when your motivation is probably at its highest) aim to complete 10 practice questions on your weakest subject and read through their explanations.

That's it - take a break.

A significant number of candidates will probably call it a day by now - I don't blame them. But unfortunately that is a way to fail. However you decide to plod on.

For your second block you complete a further 10 practice questions on your second weakest subject and read through their explanations. If your motivation wavers during any of these two blocks and the allure of that Xbox is just too great then I suggest reading a completely different topic just to reset things a little. Then take another break.

By this time it's getting late. You congratulate yourself but realise you still have one more block. The good news is that this is the block that takes the least effort and willpower on your part. Sit back, open up *Pastest* and watch one of the lectures on either of the topics you are least confident in. Try not to fall asleep.

Studying for 2 hours per day does not sound like much but it quickly adds up if you are consistent. Most candidates are unable to study for even 2 hours per day and this is reflected on the low pass rate. Nobody likes to study but if you can push through that barrier and delay gratification in the form of that Xbox then you will be rewarded.

The concept is very similar when trying to lose weight. Very few people have the motivation to run for 2 hours on the treadmill whereas variety in the form of circuit training makes things more interesting and far less mundane.

This concept should also be used during your weekends off. When your motivation is highest during the mornings you should try to get through as many practice questions in your weakest areas as possible. If your willpower weakens during this, switch to different specialties or reading materials. When you are at your absolute lowest (or feeling suicidal) then strategically use those lectures.

Have a coffee or five.

Stay motivated and keep your chin up - remember that this is only temporary!

# Logistics

When I passed parts I and II written, I was on CT1 elderly and acute medicine rotations respectively with full rotas. If you find yourself in this predicament, you will still find the time to study after work if you are dedicated enough!

Some of my more fortunate colleagues did not have on calls for a period of 3 months (due to banding issues) and used this time to focus on their exam preparation. Although there hasn't been a formal study, it's safe to assume that those with fewer on-calls were more successful in the exam and also in keeping their sanity!

If you do have a graceful period with no on-calls, ensure you use the time to actually study.

Another logistical issue to consider is whether you wish to use your annual leave strategically. Some trusts will offer you several days before the exam for travel and last minute preparation. You can increase your advantage even further by setting 1 or 2 weeks of your annual leave to coincide with the lead up to the exam.

This will require discipline and organisation skills on your part but is well worth the consideration. Remember to book study and annual leave early as many of your colleagues may be looking to do the same.

# Day of your exam

You will probably have a different pre-exam ritual but my rule was always to stop studying two days prior to the exam. You will find a lot of candidates opening their books in the waiting hall prior to the exam but I was never convinced that last minute cramming helped.

If you adopt the more relaxed approach then remember to keep yourself occupied! There is nothing worse than trying to relax but ending up ruminating
(or worse, having nightmares) about the upcoming horror. Instead, forget about the exam - easier said than done of course - take a walk, go to the cinema or spend time with your loved ones.

On the day, wake up early and give yourself plenty of time to find the venue.

Settle down. If your exam hall is far away or takes more than 30 minutes to reach then I suggest staying at a fancy hotel the night before. You should do anything that makes your experience easier.

Six hours is a very long time to stay concentrated for and that is one of the reasons why I prefer not to do last minute cramming in the waiting hall. Silly errors as a result of exhaustion would offset the odd mark you would gain from last minute revision anyway.

Keep well hydrated in the morning and make sure you use the bathroom prior to entering the exam hall. You should avoid coffee (unless you really need it for paper 2) and avoid over-hydrating as you will distract your thought process by going to the bathroom.

During the break in between papers, have a light lunch, preferably with candidates who do not discuss questions. Again many candidates will be doing practice questions and fitting in last minute revision. Unless you have superhuman concentration I recommend you do the opposite.

During the two papers, begin with the questions you are most confident with. Then return to the difficult ones and try to make an educated guess. Never leave questions blank because there is no negative marking. With BOF questions it is normally possible to eliminate a couple of wrong answers.

My last tip is to have a plan for if you finish early. Although this is unlikely to happen in part II written, finishing with time to spare is common in part I. I would recommend skim-reading all the questions again and ensuring your answers have all been transcribed correctly. I remember picking up two transcription errors in my part I exam this way.

# Failing - What Next?

The current UK trainee pass rate for MRCP Part 1 is an abysmal 50.4% so don't beat yourself up too much if you're finding it difficult. If you include all candidates, the picture is even more grim and our collective pass rate falls to 42.1%. One thing for sure is that failing MRCP Part 1 is quite common unfortunately, and in some cases several times.

If you're a UK medical graduate, the statistics above tell us your chances of passing are a coin-flip. But we know statistics can be very misleading. The pass rate can easily be skewed towards the right by some very high achievers that diet or conversely left by candidates who are only attempting MRCP Part 1 as a box-ticking exercise for CT1 applications.

Regardless of your current circumstances, here's what you should do if you find yourself failing MRCP Part 1.

Firstly, I know I know, after a 6-hour exam, the last thing you want to do is to sit down and reflect on what the hell happened! But stay disciplined, grab yourself a coffee and at least *consider* the specialty or specialties that really let you down.

Confirm this when you get your exam result three weeks later as MRCPUK usually send out a specialty breakdown that looks something like this:

| | |
|---|---|
| Cardiology | 59 |
| Clinical Haematology & Oncology | 20 |
| Clinical Pharmacology, Therapeutics & Toxicology | 54 |
| Clinical Sciences | 20 |
| Dermatology | 64 |
| Endocrinology | 45 |
| Geriatric Medicine | 90 |
| Gastroenterology | 50 |
| Infectious Diseases & GUM | 60 |
| Neurology | 45 |
| Nephrology | 48 |
| Ophthalmology | 0 |
| Psychiatry | 70 |
| Respiratory Medicine | 40 |
| Rheumatology | 40 |

At first glance, that score isn't terrible – could it maybe even scrape a pass? Unfortunately it doesn't.

When we examine the score a little more closely, we realise that the 90% mark we're really proud about for geriatrics is only worth about 1.5% of the entire exam! The key is to understand that geriatrics is only worth 4 out of the 200 marks available in the exam. The other piece of bad news is that our low score in clinical sciences actually cost us 10% of the entire exam.

It's natural to read and work on subjects you're already strong at but try and stay disciplined.

The specialty that has the most impact on your score and the one that is your weakest subject should be the target of your focussed study if you find yourself failing MRCP

Part 1. Then focus your efforts on your second weakest and the one that impacts secondarily on your *total score* and so on.

That means that using the above example, I would focus a lot more effort on clinical sciences, haematology/oncology, respiratory, rheumatology and maybe ophthalmology before attempting the exam again.

The next step is to decide when you would reapply. Assuming you've worked relatively hard for your initial attempt, I would always recommend immediately booking yourself onto the exam at the next earliest opportunity.

Just like a driving test, it would be wise to continue with driving lessons and book another test immediately. The longer you wait without driving, the less likely you are of passing the next time round.

The only caveat, of course, is if you were completely unprepared on your initial attempt. In that case I would perhaps delay it until the diet after.

30919274R00023

Printed in Great Britain
by Amazon